EASY ENDOMORPH DIET COOKBOOK FOR BEGINNERS

How To Customize Your Diet For Endomorphic Success + Delicious And Nutrient-Dense Recipes For Endomorphs

DR. LONDYN DELANEY

Table of Contents

Introductory

Understanding endomorph body types involves recognizing certain physical and metabolic characteristics. Endomorphs typically have a softer, rounder body shape with a higher percentage of body fat. Key characteristics include:

• **Body Shape**: Endomorphs tend to have a rounder physique with a wider waist and hips. They may have a larger bone structure and thicker joints.

• **Fat Distribution**: Fat tends to accumulate more in the abdomen, thighs, and hips rather than evenly distributed throughout the body.

• **Metabolism**: Endomorphs often have a slower metabolism compared to ectomorphs (leaner body type) and may find it easier to gain weight, both muscle and fat, and harder to lose weight.

• **Muscle Mass**: Endomorphs can often gain muscle mass relatively easily, which can be advantageous for strength training and bodybuilding.

• **Nutritional Considerations**: They may be more sensitive to carbohydrate intake and insulin levels, potentially requiring a diet that focuses on balanced macronutrients and portion control.

• **Exercise Recommendations**: Endomorphs tend to benefit from a combination of resistance training (to build muscle) and cardiovascular exercise (to support weight management).

It's important to note that while these characteristics describe typical endomorph traits, individuals may vary widely. Body types exist on a spectrum, and many people exhibit a combination of characteristics from different body types. Therefore, personalized approaches to diet, exercise, and lifestyle are essential for achieving health and fitness goals regardless of body type.

CHAPTER ONE
How Diet Impacts Endomorphs

Diet plays a crucial role in impacting endomorphs due to their tendency to store fat more easily and have a slower metabolism compared to other body types. Here are key considerations for how diet can affect endomorphs:

• **Caloric Intake**: Endomorphs typically need to be mindful of their caloric intake because they are more prone to weight gain. Consuming excess calories, especially from refined sugars and high-fat foods, can contribute to further fat accumulation.

• **Macronutrient Balance**: A balanced diet is important for endomorphs, focusing on moderate carbohydrates, lean proteins, and healthy fats. Carbohydrates should come from sources like whole grains, fruits, and vegetables rather than refined sugars and processed foods.

• **Protein**: Protein is crucial for muscle maintenance and growth, which can help boost metabolism and support weight management in endomorphs. Lean sources of protein such as poultry, fish, legumes, and tofu are beneficial.

• **Fiber**: Including plenty of fiber in the diet helps with satiety and can aid in regulating blood sugar levels, which is particularly important for endomorphs who may be sensitive to insulin.

• **Meal Timing and Frequency**: Eating smaller, frequent meals throughout the day can help regulate metabolism and prevent overeating. Avoiding large meals or excessive snacking can assist in managing weight.

• **Hydration**: Drinking an adequate amount of water is important for overall health and can support metabolism and digestion, which are beneficial for endomorphs.

• **Nutrient Density**: Opt for nutrient-dense foods that provide essential vitamins and minerals without excess calories. This includes vegetables, fruits, whole grains, and lean proteins.

• **Portion Control**: Endomorphs may need to pay attention to portion sizes to avoid overeating, especially of calorie-dense foods.

• **Avoiding Trigger Foods**: Some endomorphs may find certain foods trigger cravings or weight gain. Identifying and limiting these foods can be helpful in managing weight and promoting overall health.

• **Consistency and Moderation**: Consistently following a balanced diet and incorporating moderate exercise is key to achieving and maintaining a healthy weight for endomorphs.

Ultimately, individualized dietary approaches based on personal preferences, health goals, and lifestyle factors are important for endomorphs, as everyone's body responds differently to various foods and eating patterns. Consulting with a registered dietitian or nutritionist can provide personalized guidance tailored to specific needs and goals.

What Is An Endomorph?

An endomorph is one of the three primary somatotypes or body types classified by American psychologist William H. Sheldon in the 1940s. Endomorphs are characterized by certain physical and metabolic traits:

• **Body Shape**: Endomorphs typically have a rounder and softer body shape. They tend to have a wider waist and hips compared to ectomorphs (lean body type) and mesomorphs (muscular body type).

• **Fat Distribution**: They have a tendency to store fat more easily, particularly in the abdomen, thighs, and hips. This distribution can give them a more "pear-shaped" or "apple-shaped" appearance.

• **Bone Structure**: Endomorphs often have a larger bone structure and thicker joints compared to ectomorphs and mesomorphs.

• **Metabolism**: Endomorphs generally have a slower metabolism, which means they may burn calories at a slower rate compared to other body types. This can make it easier for them to gain weight, both muscle and fat, and harder to lose weight.

• **Muscle Mass**: Despite their tendency to store fat, endomorphs can often gain muscle mass relatively easily with appropriate strength training exercises.

• **Diet and Exercise**: Endomorphs may need to be more careful with their diet, focusing on balanced nutrition and portion control to manage weight effectively. They typically benefit from a combination of resistance training and cardiovascular exercise to support weight management and overall health.

It's important to note that somatotypes are a theoretical classification and most individuals do not fit perfectly into one category. Many people exhibit characteristics of multiple somatotypes to varying degrees. Therefore, while endomorphs may have certain predispositions, personalized approaches to diet, exercise, and lifestyle are crucial for achieving and maintaining health and fitness goals.

Metabolism And Energy Balance

Metabolism and energy balance play crucial roles in how our bodies function and maintain weight. Here are the key concepts related to metabolism and energy balance:

Metabolism:

- **Definition**: Metabolism refers to all the chemical processes that occur within the body to maintain life, including converting food into energy and building or repairing tissues.

- **Basal Metabolic Rate (BMR)**: BMR is the amount of energy (calories) your body needs to maintain basic physiological functions at rest, such as breathing, circulating blood, and maintaining body temperature.

Factors Affecting Metabolism:

- **Body Composition**: Muscle tissue burns more calories than fat tissue, so individuals with more muscle mass tend to have a higher metabolism.

• **Age**: Metabolism generally slows with age, primarily due to loss of muscle mass and hormonal changes.

• **Gender**: Men usually have a higher BMR than women because they tend to have more muscle mass and lower body fat percentages.

• **Genetics**: Some individuals may inherit a faster or slower metabolism from their parents.

• **Hormones**: Thyroid hormones and other hormones can influence metabolism.

• **Activity Level**: Physical activity and exercise increase metabolism, both during the activity and afterward as the body repairs and builds muscle.

Energy Balance:

• **Definition**: Energy balance is the relationship between the energy (calories) you consume through food and beverages and the energy your body expends through metabolism and physical activity.

• **Caloric Intake**: Consuming more calories than your body needs for energy expenditure leads to weight gain because the excess calories are stored as fat.

Caloric Expenditure:

• **Basal Metabolic Rate (BMR)**: Accounts for about 60-75% of total daily energy expenditure (TDEE).

• **Physical Activity**: Including exercise and non-exercise activity thermogenesis (NEAT), which varies widely between individuals.

• **Thermic Effect of Food**: The energy used by the body to digest, absorb, and metabolize food, accounting for about 10% of TDEE.

Energy Balance Equation:

Energy Balance=Calories Consumed−Calories Expended\text{Energy Balance} = \text{Calories Consumed} - \text{Calories Expended}Energy Balance=Calories Consumed−Calories Expended

• **Positive Energy Balance**: Consuming more calories than you expend leads to weight gain.

• **Negative Energy Balance**: Consuming fewer calories than you expend leads to weight loss.

• **Neutral Energy Balance**: Consuming an equal amount of calories to what you expend leads to weight maintenance.

Understanding metabolism and energy balance is crucial for managing weight and overall health. Tailoring caloric intake and physical activity to individual needs and goals can help achieve and maintain a healthy weight over time.

CHAPTER TWO
Key Nutritional Goals For Endomorphs

For endomorphs, who tend to have a slower metabolism and are more prone to storing fat, setting specific nutritional goals can help support weight management and overall health. Here are key nutritional goals tailored for endomorphs:

Caloric Intake Control:

• **Goal**: Aim to consume an appropriate amount of calories that align with your energy expenditure to avoid excess weight gain.

• **Strategy**: Calculate your Basal Metabolic Rate (BMR) and Total Daily Energy Expenditure (TDEE) to determine your daily calorie needs. Aim for a slight caloric deficit (usually 10-20% below TDEE) if weight loss is a goal.

Macronutrient Balance:

• **Goal**: Focus on a balanced intake of carbohydrates, proteins, and fats to support energy levels, muscle maintenance, and overall health.

Strategy:

• **Carbohydrates**: Choose complex carbohydrates (e.g., whole grains, fruits, vegetables) over refined sugars and processed foods to help regulate blood sugar levels and provide sustained energy.

• **Proteins**: Include lean protein sources (e.g., chicken, fish, tofu, legumes) to support muscle maintenance and metabolism.

• **Fats**: Opt for healthy fats (e.g., avocados, nuts, olive oil) in moderation to support hormone production and satiety.

Meal Timing and Frequency:

• **Goal**: Aim for regular, balanced meals and snacks to regulate metabolism and prevent overeating.

• **Strategy**: Consider spreading meals throughout the day (e.g., 3 main meals and 1-2 snacks) to maintain energy levels and prevent excessive hunger that can lead to poor food choices.

Fiber and Nutrient Density:

• **Goal**: Choose nutrient-dense foods that provide essential vitamins, minerals, and fiber without excessive calories.

• **Strategy**: Prioritize vegetables, fruits, whole grains, and lean proteins to promote satiety, support digestive health, and maintain overall well-being.

Hydration:

- **Goal**: Stay adequately hydrated to support metabolism, digestion, and overall health.

- **Strategy**: Drink plenty of water throughout the day and limit sugary beverages and alcohol, which can contribute unnecessary calories.

Portion Control and Mindful Eating:

- **Goal**: Practice portion control and mindful eating to avoid overeating and manage calorie intake.

- **Strategy**: Use smaller plates, pay attention to hunger cues, and eat slowly to allow time for feelings of fullness to develop.

Exercise and Physical Activity:

- **Goal**: Incorporate regular exercise to support metabolism, muscle development, and overall health.

- **Strategy**: Include a combination of resistance training (to build muscle) and aerobic exercise (to burn calories) for optimal weight management and fitness.

By focusing on these key nutritional goals, endomorphs can create a balanced and sustainable eating plan that supports their unique metabolism and helps achieve their health and fitness objectives. Adjustments may be necessary based on individual responses and goals, so consulting with a registered dietitian or nutritionist can provide personalized guidance.

Planning Your Endomorph Diet

Planning a diet tailored for an endomorph involves focusing on nutrient balance, calorie control, and supporting metabolic health. Here's a structured approach to help you plan your diet effectively:

1. Calculate Your Caloric Needs:

Determine your Basal Metabolic Rate (BMR) and Total Daily Energy Expenditure (TDEE) to understand how many calories you need each day. This helps establish whether you should aim for weight maintenance, weight loss, or weight gain.

Adjust your caloric intake based on your goals:

• **Weight Loss**: Create a moderate caloric deficit (typically 10-20% below TDEE).

• **Weight Maintenance**: Consume calories that match your TDEE.

• **Weight Gain**: Gradually increase your caloric intake above your TDEE, focusing on muscle gain rather than fat accumulation.

2. Focus on Balanced Macronutrients:

• **Carbohydrates**: Choose complex carbohydrates such as whole grains (brown rice, quinoa), fruits, and vegetables. Limit simple carbohydrates like sugary snacks and refined grains.

• **Proteins**: Include lean protein sources such as chicken breast, turkey, fish, tofu, legumes, and low-fat dairy. Protein helps with muscle maintenance and can support metabolism.

• **Fats**: Opt for healthy fats like avocados, nuts, seeds, and olive oil. These fats provide essential fatty acids and support hormone production.

3. Meal Planning:

• **Regular Meals**: Plan balanced meals throughout the day to maintain steady energy levels and prevent overeating.

• **Portion Control**: Use smaller plates and practice mindful eating to control portions and avoid consuming excess calories.

• **Snacking**: Incorporate healthy snacks like yogurt with fruits, nuts, or vegetables with hummus to manage hunger between meals.

4. Nutrient Density:

• Choose nutrient-dense foods that provide essential vitamins, minerals, and fiber without excessive calories. Prioritize vegetables, fruits, lean proteins, and whole grains.

5. Hydration:

• Drink plenty of water throughout the day to support metabolism, digestion, and overall health. Limit sugary drinks and alcohol, as they can add unnecessary calories.

6. Exercise and Physical Activity:

• Incorporate a combination of resistance training (weightlifting, bodyweight exercises) and cardiovascular exercise (walking, running, swimming) to support metabolism, muscle development, and weight management.

• Aim for at least 150 minutes of moderate-intensity aerobic activity per week, along with muscle-strengthening activities on two or more days a week.

7. Monitor Progress and Adjust:

• Regularly monitor your weight, body measurements, and how you feel. Adjust your diet and exercise plan as needed to maintain progress toward your goals.

• Consider consulting with a registered dietitian or nutritionist for personalized guidance based on your specific needs, preferences, and health goals.

By planning your diet around these principles—calorie control, balanced macronutrients, nutrient density, hydration, and physical activity—you can create a sustainable and effective eating plan that supports your health as an endomorph. Adjustments may be necessary based on individual responses and goals, so stay flexible and proactive in your approach.

CHAPTER THREE
Foods To Include In Your Diet

When planning a diet for an endomorph, it's important to focus on nutrient-dense foods that support metabolism, promote satiety, and provide essential nutrients without excessive calories. Here's a list of foods that are beneficial for endomorphs to include in their diet:

1. Lean Proteins:

- Chicken breast
- Turkey breast
- Lean cuts of beef or pork
- Fish (salmon, trout, tuna)
- Shellfish (shrimp, crab)
- Tofu and tempeh
- Legumes (beans, lentils, chickpeas)

2. Whole Grains:

- Quinoa

- Brown rice
- Oats (steel-cut or rolled)
- Whole wheat pasta
- Barley
- Buckwheat
- Whole grain bread and wraps

3. Vegetables:

- Leafy greens (spinach, kale, Swiss chard)
- Cruciferous vegetables (broccoli, cauliflower, Brussels sprouts)
- Bell peppers
- Tomatoes
- Cucumber
- Zucchini
- Carrots

4. Fruits:

- Berries (strawberries, blueberries, raspberries)

- Apples

- Oranges

- Bananas

- Kiwi

- Pineapple

- Grapefruit

5. Healthy Fats:

- Avocados

- Nuts (almonds, walnuts, cashews)

- Seeds (chia seeds, flaxseeds, pumpkin seeds)

- Olive oil

- Coconut oil (use in moderation)

- Fatty fish (salmon, mackerel)

6. Dairy or Dairy Alternatives:

- Greek yogurt (plain, low-fat or non-fat)

- Cottage cheese (low-fat)

- Milk (low-fat or plant-based alternatives like almond or soy milk)
- Cheese (in moderation, opt for lower-fat varieties)

7. Legumes and Beans:

- Black beans
- Kidney beans
- Lentils
- Chickpeas
- Edamame

8. Other Foods:

- Eggs (boiled, scrambled, or as omelets)
- Tofu and tempeh (plant-based protein sources)
- Herbs and spices (use to add flavor without extra calories)
- Dark chocolate (in moderation, at least 70% cocoa)

Tips for Incorporation:

• **Balanced Meals**: Combine lean proteins, whole grains, and vegetables for balanced meals that provide sustained energy and fullness.

• **Snacks**: Opt for fruits, nuts, yogurt, or vegetable sticks with hummus for nutritious snacks between meals.

• **Hydration**: Drink plenty of water throughout the day and consider herbal teas or infused water for added variety.

• **Cooking Methods**: Use healthy cooking methods like grilling, baking, steaming, or sautéing with minimal oil to keep meals nutritious and lower in calories.

By incorporating these foods into your diet, you can support your metabolism, manage weight effectively, and ensure your body receives essential nutrients for overall health as an endomorph. Adjust portion sizes and meal timing based on your individual caloric needs and goals for optimal results.

Foods To Limit Or Avoid

For endomorphs, it's important to be mindful of foods that can contribute excess calories, sugar, unhealthy fats, and lack sufficient nutrients. Here are foods to limit or avoid in your diet:

1. Refined Carbohydrates:

- White bread
- White rice
- Pastries and baked goods (cakes, cookies, doughnuts)
- Sugary cereals
- Sugary drinks (soda, sweetened coffee drinks, energy drinks)

2. Sugary Foods and Sweets:

- Candy
- Chocolate bars with high sugar content
- Ice cream and frozen desserts

- Syrups and sugary toppings (e.g., maple syrup, honey in large quantities)

3. Processed and High-Fat Meats:

- Processed meats (sausage, bacon, deli meats)
- Fatty cuts of beef and pork (ribeye, T-bone steak)
- Fried meats (fried chicken, breaded meats)

4. Fried Foods and Fast Food:

- French fries
- Fried chicken
- Fast food burgers and sandwiches
- Breaded and fried appetizers (mozzarella sticks, onion rings)

5. High-Fat Dairy Products:

- Full-fat cheese (cheddar, mozzarella)
- Cream cheese

- Full-fat yogurt and sour cream

- Ice cream and rich desserts made with heavy cream

6. Sugary Sauces and Dressings:

- Barbecue sauce

- Teriyaki sauce

- Sweetened salad dressings

- Ketchup and other condiments high in sugar

7. Alcohol:

- Beer

- Sweetened cocktails

- Wine coolers

- Sugary mixed drinks and cocktails

8. Snack Foods and Processed Snacks:

- Potato chips

- Crackers with added sugars or fats

- Packaged snack cakes and pastries

- Microwave popcorn with added butter or caramel

Tips for Managing:

• **Read Labels**: Check food labels for added sugars, unhealthy fats (saturated and trans fats), and high-calorie content.

• **Portion Control**: If you choose to consume these foods occasionally, practice moderation and be mindful of portion sizes.

• **Healthy Alternatives**: Look for healthier alternatives or make homemade versions of favorite snacks and treats using healthier ingredients.

• **Meal Planning**: Plan meals and snacks ahead of time to avoid impulse eating of unhealthy foods.

- **Hydration**: Drink water or unsweetened beverages instead of sugary drinks and limit alcohol intake.

By limiting these foods in your diet, you can better manage calorie intake, support healthy weight management, and promote overall well-being as an endomorph.

Focus on a balanced diet rich in nutrient-dense foods while minimizing foods that provide empty calories and little nutritional value.

CHAPTER FOUR
Sample Meal Plans

Creating a sample meal plan for an endomorph involves balancing macronutrients, controlling portion sizes, and choosing nutrient-dense foods to support metabolism and weight management. Here are two sample meal plans for a day:

Sample Meal Plan 1:

Breakfast:

Greek Yogurt Parfait

- Greek yogurt (plain, low-fat or non-fat): 1 cup
- Mixed berries (strawberries, blueberries): 1/2 cup
- Granola (low-sugar, whole grain): 1/4 cup
- Honey (optional): drizzle

Snack:

Apple with Almond Butter

- Apple: 1 medium
- Almond butter (unsweetened): 2 tablespoons

Lunch:

Grilled Chicken Salad

- Grilled chicken breast: 4 oz
- Mixed greens (spinach, kale): 2 cups
- Cherry tomatoes: 1/2 cup
- Cucumber slices: 1/2 cup
- Olive oil and vinegar dressing: 2 tablespoons

Snack:

Carrots and Hummus

- Baby carrots: 1 cup
- Hummus (low-fat): 2 tablespoons

Dinner:

Baked Salmon with Quinoa and Vegetables

- Salmon fillet: 4 oz
- Quinoa (cooked): 1/2 cup
- Steamed broccoli: 1 cup
- Lemon wedge for squeezing over salmon

Evening Snack (Optional):

Greek Yogurt with Berries

- Greek yogurt (plain, low-fat or non-fat): 1/2 cup
- Mixed berries: 1/2 cup

Sample Meal Plan 2:

Breakfast:

Oatmeal with Fruit and Nuts

- Rolled oats (cooked): 1/2 cup
- Sliced banana: 1/2
- Almonds (sliced): 1 tablespoon
- Cinnamon (optional): sprinkle

Snack:

Protein Smoothie

- Protein powder (whey or plant-based): 1 scoop
- Spinach: 1 cup
- Frozen berries (mixed): 1/2 cup
- Unsweetened almond milk: 1 cup

Lunch:

Turkey and Avocado Wrap

- Whole grain wrap: 1 large
- Sliced turkey breast: 3 oz

- Avocado (sliced): 1/4

- Mixed greens: 1 cup

- Mustard or low-fat mayo: 1 tablespoon

Snack:

Greek Yogurt with Nuts

- Greek yogurt (plain, low-fat or non-fat): 1 cup

- Mixed nuts (almonds, walnuts): 1/4 cup

Dinner:

Stir-Fried Tofu with Vegetables and Brown Rice

- Firm tofu (cubed): 4 oz

- Mixed stir-fry vegetables (bell peppers, broccoli, carrots): 1 cup

- Brown rice (cooked): 1/2 cup

- Stir-fry sauce (low-sodium): 2 tablespoons

Evening Snack (Optional):

Cottage Cheese with Pineapple

- Cottage cheese (low-fat): 1/2 cup
- Pineapple chunks (fresh or canned in juice): 1/2 cup

Tips for Meal Planning:

• **Variety**: Incorporate a variety of foods from different food groups to ensure you get a wide range of nutrients.

• **Portion Control**: Be mindful of portion sizes to avoid overeating, especially with calorie-dense foods.

• **Hydration**: Drink water throughout the day to stay hydrated and support metabolism.

• **Preparation**: Plan and prepare meals and snacks ahead of time to avoid unhealthy food choices.

• **Adjustments**: Modify portion sizes and food choices based on your caloric needs and dietary preferences.

These sample meal plans provide a foundation for balanced nutrition for endomorphs. Adjust quantities and specific foods based on individual preferences, dietary restrictions, and goals. For personalized guidance, consider consulting with a registered dietitian or nutritionist.

Quick And Easy Recipes For Endomorphs

For individuals who identify as endomorphs (those who tend to store more fat and have a rounded physique), quick and easy recipes should focus on balanced meals that provide sustained energy without excessive carbohydrates or unhealthy fats. Here are some ideas:

Breakfast:

Greek Yogurt Parfait:

• Layer Greek yogurt with fresh berries, a drizzle of honey or maple syrup, and a sprinkle of nuts or seeds.

Avocado Toast:

• Mash avocado on whole grain toast, top with a poached egg, and sprinkle with salt, pepper, and a dash of hot sauce.

Lunch:

Grilled Chicken Salad:

• Grill chicken breast and serve over mixed greens with cherry tomatoes, cucumber slices, and a light vinaigrette dressing.

Quinoa and Vegetable Stir-Fry:

• Sauté mixed vegetables (like bell peppers, broccoli, and snap peas) with cooked quinoa, soy sauce, and a touch of sesame oil.

Dinner:

Baked Salmon with Roasted Vegetables:

• Season salmon fillets with herbs and lemon, then bake until flaky. Serve with roasted sweet potatoes and steamed broccoli.

Turkey and Quinoa Stuffed Peppers:

• Fill bell peppers with a mixture of cooked ground turkey, quinoa, diced tomatoes, and spices. Bake until peppers are tender.

Snacks:

Smoothie Bowl:

• Blend spinach, frozen berries, Greek yogurt, and a splash of almond milk. Top with granola and chia seeds.

Apple Slices with Almond Butter:

• Slice apples and dip in almond butter for a satisfying snack.

Tips for Endomorphs:

• **Balanced Macros:** Aim for meals that are balanced with lean protein, healthy fats, and complex carbohydrates (like whole grains and vegetables).

• **Portion Control:** Pay attention to portion sizes to manage calorie intake.

- **Regular Exercise:** Combine these meals with regular physical activity to support metabolism and overall health.

These recipes are designed to provide nutritious options that support weight management and sustained energy levels, which can be beneficial for individuals with an endomorphic body type. Adjust portion sizes and ingredients based on personal preferences and dietary needs.

Slow-Cooker Chicken & White Bean Stew Recipes

Here's a simple Slow-Cooker Chicken & White Bean Stew recipe for you:

Ingredients:

- 1.5 lbs (about 680g) boneless, skinless chicken breasts or thighs, cut into cubes
- 2 cans (15 oz each) white beans (such as cannellini or great Northern), drained and rinsed
- 1 onion, finely chopped
- 3 cloves garlic, minced
- 2 carrots, peeled and sliced
- 2 celery stalks, sliced
- 1 can (14.5 oz) diced tomatoes, undrained
- 4 cups chicken broth
- 1 teaspoon dried thyme
- 1 teaspoon dried rosemary

- 1 bay leaf

- Salt and pepper, to taste

- Fresh parsley, chopped (for garnish)

Instructions:

• **Prep Ingredients**: Chop the onion, mince the garlic, peel and slice the carrots, and slice the celery stalks.

• **Combine Ingredients in Slow Cooker**: Place the cubed chicken, drained and rinsed white beans, chopped onion, minced garlic, sliced carrots, sliced celery, diced tomatoes (with their juices), chicken broth, dried thyme, dried rosemary, bay leaf, salt, and pepper into the slow cooker. Stir well to combine.

• **Cook**: Cover and cook on low for 6-8 hours, or on high for 3-4 hours, until the chicken is cooked through and vegetables are tender.

- **Adjust Seasoning**: Taste and adjust seasoning with salt and pepper if needed.

- **Serve**: Discard the bay leaf. Ladle the stew into bowls and garnish with chopped fresh parsley.

- **Enjoy**: Serve hot, optionally with crusty bread or over rice.

This recipe is hearty, flavorful, and perfect for a comforting meal. Adjust the seasoning and thickness of the stew to your preference by adding more broth or letting it reduce further during cooking.

Creamy Chicken, Brussels Sprouts & Mushrooms One-Pot Pasta Recipes

Here's a recipe for Creamy Chicken, Brussels Sprouts & Mushrooms One-Pot Pasta:

Ingredients:

- 1 lb (about 450g) boneless, skinless chicken breasts, cut into cubes
- 8 oz (225g) Brussels sprouts, trimmed and halved
- 8 oz (225g) mushrooms (cremini or button), sliced
- 1 onion, finely chopped
- 3 cloves garlic, minced
- 8 oz (225g) linguine or fettuccine pasta
- 4 cups chicken broth
- 1 cup heavy cream
- 1/2 cup grated Parmesan cheese
- 2 tablespoons olive oil
- 1 teaspoon dried thyme
- Salt and pepper, to taste
- Fresh parsley, chopped (for garnish)

Instructions:

• **Sauté Chicken and Vegetables**: In a large pot or deep skillet, heat 1 tablespoon of olive oil over medium-high heat. Add the cubed chicken and season with salt and pepper. Cook until chicken is browned and cooked through, about 5-6 minutes. Remove chicken from the pot and set aside.

• **Cook Vegetables**: In the same pot, add another tablespoon of olive oil if needed. Add the chopped onion and cook until softened, about 3-4 minutes. Add minced garlic, Brussels sprouts, and mushrooms. Cook for another 4-5 minutes until vegetables are slightly softened.

• **Add Pasta and Broth**: Add the linguine (or fettuccine) pasta to the pot, breaking it in half if necessary to fit. Pour in the chicken broth and dried thyme. Bring to a boil, then reduce heat to medium-low. Cover and simmer, stirring occasionally, for about 10-12 minutes, or until pasta is al dente and most of the liquid is absorbed.

• **Add Cream and Cheese**: Stir in the heavy cream and grated Parmesan cheese until well combined. Add the cooked chicken back into the pot. Cook for an additional 2-3 minutes, stirring occasionally, until everything is heated through and the sauce has thickened slightly.

• **Adjust Seasoning and Serve**: Taste and adjust seasoning with salt and pepper if needed. Remove from heat. Garnish with chopped fresh parsley before serving.

• **Enjoy**: Serve hot, garnished with extra Parmesan cheese if desired. Enjoy your creamy one-pot pasta with chicken, Brussels sprouts, and mushrooms!

This dish is creamy, comforting, and packed with delicious flavors from the chicken and vegetables. It's perfect for a satisfying meal any day of the week.

Chipotle Chicken Quinoa Burrito Bowl Recipes

Here's a recipe for a Chipotle Chicken Quinoa Burrito Bowl:

Ingredients:

For the Chipotle Chicken:

- 1 lb (about 450g) boneless, skinless chicken breasts, thinly sliced
- 2 tablespoons olive oil
- 1 chipotle pepper in adobo sauce, minced (plus 1 tablespoon adobo sauce)
- 1 teaspoon ground cumin
- 1 teaspoon chili powder
- 1/2 teaspoon paprika
- Salt and pepper, to taste

For the Quinoa:

- 1 cup quinoa, rinsed
- 2 cups chicken broth or water

- Salt, to taste

For the Burrito Bowl:

- 1 can (15 oz) black beans, drained and rinsed
- 1 cup corn kernels (fresh, canned, or frozen)
- 1 red bell pepper, diced
- 1 avocado, sliced
- 1 cup cherry tomatoes, halved
- Fresh cilantro, chopped (for garnish)
- Lime wedges (for serving)

Optional toppings:

- Shredded lettuce or mixed greens
- Sour cream or Greek yogurt
- Salsa or pico de gallo
- Shredded cheese

Instructions:

Prepare the Chipotle Chicken:

• In a bowl, combine olive oil, minced chipotle pepper with adobo sauce, cumin, chili powder, paprika, salt, and pepper.

• Add the sliced chicken breast to the bowl and toss until well coated. Marinate for at least 15 minutes.

Cook the Quinoa:

• In a saucepan, combine quinoa and chicken broth (or water) with a pinch of salt. Bring to a boil, then reduce heat to low, cover, and simmer for about 15 minutes, or until quinoa is cooked and liquid is absorbed. Fluff with a fork and set aside.

Cook the Chipotle Chicken:

• Heat a large skillet over medium-high heat. Add the marinated chicken slices and cook for 5-6 minutes, stirring occasionally, until chicken is cooked through and nicely browned. Remove from heat and set aside.

Prepare the Burrito Bowl Ingredients:

• In the same skillet (if desired, for fewer dishes), add a little olive oil if needed and sauté the diced red bell pepper until slightly softened, about 3-4 minutes.

• Add the black beans and corn kernels to the skillet. Cook for another 2-3 minutes until heated through.

Assemble the Burrito Bowl:

• Divide cooked quinoa among serving bowls. Top with the chipotle chicken, sautéed black beans and corn mixture, sliced avocado, cherry tomatoes, and any optional toppings you prefer (lettuce, sour cream, salsa, cheese).

Garnish and Serve:

• Sprinkle chopped cilantro over the bowls. Serve with lime wedges on the side for squeezing over the bowl before eating.

Enjoy:

• Mix everything together in the bowl before eating to enjoy the flavors. This Chipotle Chicken Quinoa Burrito Bowl is nutritious, flavorful, and customizable to suit your taste preferences.

Middle Eastern Chicken & Chickpea Stew

Middle Eastern Chicken & Chickpea Stew is a delicious and comforting dish. Here's a recipe you can try:

Ingredients:

- 1.5 lbs (about 680g) boneless, skinless chicken thighs or breasts, cut into bite-sized pieces
- 1 onion, finely chopped
- 3 cloves garlic, minced
- 1 teaspoon ground cumin
- 1 teaspoon ground coriander
- 1/2 teaspoon ground turmeric
- 1/2 teaspoon ground cinnamon
- 1/4 teaspoon ground cloves
- 1/4 teaspoon cayenne pepper (adjust to taste)
- 1 can (15 oz) chickpeas (garbanzo beans), drained and rinsed

- 1 can (14.5 oz) diced tomatoes
- 1 cup chicken broth
- 1/4 cup chopped fresh cilantro, plus more for garnish
- 1/4 cup chopped fresh parsley, plus more for garnish
- Juice of 1 lemon
- Salt and pepper, to taste
- Olive oil, for cooking

Instructions:

• **Sauté Chicken:** Heat olive oil in a large pot or Dutch oven over medium-high heat. Add the chopped onion and cook until softened, about 5 minutes. Add minced garlic and cook for another 1-2 minutes until fragrant.

• **Add Spices:** Add ground cumin, ground coriander, ground turmeric, ground cinnamon, ground cloves, and cayenne pepper to the pot. Stir well to coat the onions and garlic with the spices.

- **Cook Chicken:** Add the chicken pieces to the pot and cook until browned on all sides, about 5-7 minutes.

- **Combine Chickpeas and Tomatoes:** Add the drained and rinsed chickpeas and diced tomatoes (with their juices) to the pot. Stir to combine.

- **Simmer:** Pour in the chicken broth. Bring the stew to a simmer, then reduce the heat to low. Cover and let it simmer gently for about 20-25 minutes, stirring occasionally, until the chicken is cooked through and tender.

- **Add Fresh Herbs and Lemon Juice:** Stir in the chopped fresh cilantro and parsley. Squeeze in the juice of one lemon. Season with salt and pepper to taste.

- **Serve:** Ladle the stew into bowls. Garnish with additional chopped cilantro and parsley if desired. Serve hot, optionally with rice or crusty bread.

• **Enjoy:** This Middle Eastern Chicken & Chickpea Stew is flavorful with warm spices and herbs, and the chickpeas add a lovely texture. It's perfect for a cozy dinner and can be easily adjusted by adding more spice or adjusting the lemon juice to your taste preferences.

Pistachio-Crusted Chicken With Warm Barley Salad Recipes

Here's a delicious recipe for Pistachio-Crusted Chicken with Warm Barley Salad:

Ingredients:

For the Pistachio-Crusted Chicken:

- 4 boneless, skinless chicken breasts
- 1 cup shelled pistachios, finely chopped or ground

- 1/2 cup breadcrumbs (preferably panko)
- 1/4 cup grated Parmesan cheese
- 1 teaspoon dried thyme
- 1/2 teaspoon garlic powder
- Salt and pepper, to taste
- 2 eggs, beaten
- Olive oil, for cooking

For the Warm Barley Salad:

- 1 cup pearl barley
- 3 cups chicken broth or water
- 1 tablespoon olive oil
- 1 small red onion, finely chopped
- 1 bell pepper (any color), diced
- 1 cup cherry tomatoes, halved
- 1/2 cup cucumber, diced
- 1/4 cup chopped fresh parsley
- Juice of 1 lemon
- Salt and pepper, to taste

Instructions:

For the Pistachio-Crusted Chicken:

• Preheat your oven to 400°F (200°C).

• In a shallow bowl or plate, combine finely chopped pistachios, breadcrumbs, grated Parmesan cheese, dried thyme, garlic powder, salt, and pepper.

• Place the beaten eggs in another shallow bowl.

• Pat dry the chicken breasts with paper towels. Dip each chicken breast into the beaten eggs, then coat with the pistachio mixture, pressing gently to adhere.

• Heat olive oil in a large oven-safe skillet over medium-high heat. Add the pistachio-crusted chicken breasts and cook for 3-4 minutes per side, until golden brown.

• Transfer the skillet to the preheated oven and bake for 15-20 minutes, or until the chicken is cooked through (internal temperature of 165°F or 74°C).

• Remove from oven and let the chicken rest for a few minutes before slicing.

For the Warm Barley Salad:

• Rinse the pearl barley under cold water. In a saucepan, bring 3 cups of chicken broth (or water) to a boil. Add the rinsed barley, reduce heat to low, cover, and simmer for about 30-35 minutes, or until barley is tender and liquid is absorbed. Remove from heat and let it sit covered for 5 minutes.

• While the barley is cooking, heat 1 tablespoon of olive oil in a skillet over medium heat. Add finely chopped red onion and diced bell pepper. Cook for 3-4 minutes until softened.

• In a large bowl, combine cooked barley, sautéed red onion and bell pepper, halved cherry tomatoes, diced cucumber, chopped fresh parsley, and lemon juice. Season with salt and pepper to taste. Toss everything together until well combined.

To Serve:

• Divide the warm barley salad among serving plates. Top each portion with slices of pistachio-crusted chicken.

• Garnish with additional chopped parsley or a sprinkle of extra pistachios if desired.

Serve immediately and enjoy this flavorful and nutritious Pistachio-Crusted Chicken with Warm Barley Salad!

Chicken & Vegetable Penne With Parsley-Walnut Pesto Recipes

Here's a delightful recipe for Chicken & Vegetable Penne with Parsley-Walnut Pesto:

Ingredients:

For the Parsley-Walnut Pesto:

- 1 cup fresh parsley leaves, packed
- 1/2 cup walnuts, toasted
- 1/4 cup grated Parmesan cheese
- 2 cloves garlic, peeled
- Juice of 1 lemon
- 1/3 cup olive oil
- Salt and pepper, to taste

For the Chicken & Vegetable Penne:

- 12 oz (340g) penne pasta
- 1 lb (about 450g) boneless, skinless chicken breasts, cut into bite-sized pieces
- 1 tablespoon olive oil
- 1 red bell pepper, thinly sliced
- 1 yellow bell pepper, thinly sliced
- 1 zucchini, halved lengthwise and thinly sliced

- 1 cup cherry tomatoes, halved
- Salt and pepper, to taste
- Grated Parmesan cheese, for serving
- Fresh parsley leaves, chopped, for garnish

Instructions:

1. Make the Parsley-Walnut Pesto:

• In a food processor, combine fresh parsley leaves, toasted walnuts, grated Parmesan cheese, garlic cloves, and lemon juice.

• Pulse until finely chopped.

• With the food processor running, slowly drizzle in the olive oil until the pesto reaches your desired consistency.

• Season with salt and pepper to taste. Set aside.

2. Cook the Penne Pasta:

• Bring a large pot of salted water to a boil. Cook the penne pasta according to package instructions until al dente. Drain and set aside, reserving about 1/2 cup of pasta water.

3. Prepare the Chicken & Vegetables:

• While the pasta is cooking, heat 1 tablespoon of olive oil in a large skillet or pan over medium-high heat.

• Add the bite-sized chicken pieces to the skillet. Season with salt and pepper. Cook, stirring occasionally, until the chicken is cooked through and nicely browned, about 5-6 minutes. Remove the chicken from the skillet and set aside.

• In the same skillet, add the sliced red bell pepper, yellow bell pepper, and zucchini. Cook, stirring occasionally, for about 4-5 minutes until the vegetables are tender-crisp.

• Add the cherry tomatoes to the skillet and cook for an additional 2 minutes until heated through.

4. Assemble the Dish:

• Return the cooked penne pasta to the skillet with the vegetables.

• Add the cooked chicken back to the skillet.

• Pour the prepared parsley-walnut pesto over the pasta, chicken, and vegetables. Toss everything together gently until well combined, adding a splash of reserved pasta water if needed to loosen the sauce.

• Heat through for 1-2 minutes, stirring gently.

5. Serve:

• Divide the Chicken & Vegetable Penne with Parsley-Walnut Pesto among serving plates.

- Garnish with grated Parmesan cheese and chopped fresh parsley leaves.

- Serve immediately and enjoy this flavorful and vibrant pasta dish!

- This recipe combines the richness of the parsley-walnut pesto with the tenderness of chicken and the freshness of seasonal vegetables, making it a perfect choice for a satisfying meal.

Honey-Mustard Chicken Tenders With Couscous & Carrots Recipes

Here's a delicious recipe for Honey-Mustard Chicken Tenders with Couscous & Carrots:

Ingredients:

For the Honey-Mustard Chicken Tenders:

- 1 lb (about 450g) chicken tenders or boneless, skinless chicken breasts cut into strips

- 1/4 cup Dijon mustard

- 2 tablespoons honey

- 2 tablespoons olive oil

- 1 tablespoon apple cider vinegar (or white wine vinegar)

- 2 cloves garlic, minced

- 1 teaspoon dried thyme (or use fresh if available)

- Salt and pepper, to taste

For the Couscous & Carrots:

- 1 cup couscous

- 1.5 cups chicken broth (or water)

- 1 tablespoon olive oil

- 1 onion, finely chopped

- 2 carrots, peeled and diced

- Salt and pepper, to taste

- Fresh parsley or cilantro, chopped (for garnish)

Instructions:

1. **Prepare the Honey-Mustard Chicken Tenders:**

- In a bowl, whisk together Dijon mustard, honey, olive oil, apple cider vinegar, minced garlic, dried thyme, salt, and pepper.

- Add the chicken tenders to the bowl and toss until evenly coated with the marinade. Cover and let marinate in the refrigerator for at least 30 minutes, or up to 4 hours for more flavor.

- Preheat the oven to 400°F (200°C). Line a baking sheet with parchment paper or foil.

- Arrange the marinated chicken tenders on the prepared baking sheet in a single layer. Bake for 15-20 minutes, or until the chicken is cooked through and golden brown. Cooking time may vary depending on the thickness of the chicken tenders.

2. Prepare the Couscous & Carrots:

• While the chicken is baking, prepare the couscous according to package instructions. Typically, bring 1.5 cups of chicken broth or water to a boil. Stir in couscous, cover, and remove from heat. Let it sit for about 5 minutes, then fluff with a fork.

• In a separate skillet, heat 1 tablespoon of olive oil over medium heat. Add finely chopped onion and diced carrots. Cook, stirring occasionally, until vegetables are tender, about 5-7 minutes. Season with salt and pepper to taste.

• Add the cooked couscous to the skillet with the vegetables. Stir gently to combine and heat through for another minute or two.

3. Serve:

• Divide the couscous and carrots among serving plates.

• Top with the honey-mustard chicken tenders.

• Garnish with chopped fresh parsley or cilantro.

• Serve immediately and enjoy this flavorful and wholesome dish!

This Honey-Mustard Chicken Tenders with Couscous & Carrots recipe is easy to prepare and provides a balanced meal with protein, grains, and vegetables, all flavored with a sweet and tangy honey-mustard marinade.

Paprika Chicken Thighs With Brussels Sprouts For Two Recipes

Here's a tasty recipe for Paprika Chicken Thighs with Brussels Sprouts for Two:

Ingredients:

- 2 bone-in, skin-on chicken thighs
- 1 tablespoon olive oil

- 1 teaspoon paprika

- 1/2 teaspoon garlic powder

- 1/2 teaspoon onion powder

- Salt and pepper, to taste

- 8 oz Brussels sprouts, trimmed and halved

- 1 tablespoon balsamic vinegar

- 1 tablespoon honey

- 1 tablespoon olive oil

- Salt and pepper, to taste

Instructions:

Prepare the Chicken Thighs:

• Preheat your oven to 400°F (200°C).

• In a small bowl, mix together paprika, garlic powder, onion powder, salt, and pepper.

• Rub the spice mixture all over the chicken thighs, ensuring they are evenly coated.

• Heat 1 tablespoon of olive oil in an oven-safe skillet over medium-high heat.

• Place the chicken thighs in the skillet, skin side down. Cook for about 5-6 minutes, until the skin is golden brown and crispy. Flip the thighs and cook for another 3-4 minutes on the other side.

• Transfer the skillet to the preheated oven. Bake for 20-25 minutes, or until the chicken thighs reach an internal temperature of 165°F (74°C) and juices run clear.

Prepare the Brussels Sprouts:

• While the chicken is baking, prepare the Brussels sprouts.

• In a bowl, whisk together balsamic vinegar, honey, and 1 tablespoon of olive oil.

• Toss the halved Brussels sprouts in the balsamic-honey mixture until well coated. Season with salt and pepper to taste.

• Spread the Brussels sprouts on a baking sheet lined with parchment paper or foil.

• Roast in the oven at 400°F (200°C) for about 15-20 minutes, or until the Brussels sprouts are tender and caramelized, shaking the pan halfway through.

Serve:

• Once the chicken thighs are cooked through and the Brussels sprouts are roasted, divide them between two plates.

• Serve the paprika chicken thighs alongside the roasted Brussels sprouts.

• Enjoy your delicious and flavorful meal for two!

This recipe combines the smoky flavor of paprika-spiced chicken thighs with the sweetness of honey-balsamic Brussels sprouts, making it a perfect meal for a cozy dinner for two. Adjust the seasoning and cooking times based on your preferences and oven behavior for the best results!

Classic Sesame Noodles With Chicken Recipes

Here's a recipe for Classic Sesame Noodles with Chicken, a delicious and satisfying dish:

Ingredients:

For the Sesame Noodles:

- 8 oz (225g) Chinese egg noodles or spaghetti
- 2 tablespoons sesame oil
- 3 tablespoons soy sauce (low sodium recommended)
- 2 tablespoons rice vinegar

- 1 tablespoon honey or brown sugar

- 1 tablespoon sesame seeds, toasted

- 2 green onions, thinly sliced

- Crushed red pepper flakes, to taste (optional)

For the Chicken:

- 1 lb (about 450g) boneless, skinless chicken breasts or thighs, cut into bite-sized pieces

- 1 tablespoon soy sauce

- 1 tablespoon hoisin sauce

- 1 tablespoon cornstarch

- 1 tablespoon vegetable oil

Optional Garnishes:

- Thinly sliced cucumber

- Shredded carrots

- Chopped cilantro or parsley

Instructions:

1. Prepare the Sesame Noodles:

• Cook the Chinese egg noodles or spaghetti according to package instructions until al dente. Drain and rinse under cold water to stop cooking. Set aside.

• In a small bowl, whisk together sesame oil, soy sauce, rice vinegar, honey or brown sugar, toasted sesame seeds, sliced green onions, and crushed red pepper flakes (if using).

• Toss the cooked noodles with the sesame sauce until well coated. Adjust seasoning to taste. Set aside.

2. Cook the Chicken:

• In a bowl, combine the chicken pieces with soy sauce, hoisin sauce, and cornstarch. Mix until the chicken is evenly coated.

• Heat vegetable oil in a large skillet or wok over medium-high heat. Add the chicken pieces in a single layer and cook for about 5-6 minutes, stirring occasionally, until browned and cooked through.

• Remove the chicken from the skillet and set aside.

3. Assemble the Dish:

• Divide the sesame noodles among serving plates.

• Top each serving with the cooked chicken pieces.

• Garnish with optional toppings such as thinly sliced cucumber, shredded carrots, and chopped cilantro or parsley.

• Serve immediately and enjoy your Classic Sesame Noodles with Chicken!

This recipe offers a perfect balance of savory sesame flavors with tender chicken and noodles. It's quick to make and can be customized with additional vegetables or garnishes to suit your preferences.

CHAPTER FIVE
Overcoming Cravings And Emotional Eating

Overcoming cravings and emotional eating can be challenging but achievable with a combination of strategies focusing on mindfulness, healthy habits, and understanding triggers. Here are some effective approaches:

1. Identify Triggers and Patterns:

• **Keep a Food Diary:** Record what you eat, when you eat, and how you feel before and after eating. This can help identify patterns and emotional triggers for eating.

• **Recognize Emotional Triggers:** Pay attention to situations, emotions (stress, boredom, sadness), or activities that prompt cravings or emotional eating episodes.

2. Develop Healthy Eating Habits:

• **Regular Meals:** Stick to regular meal times and avoid skipping meals, which can lead to overeating later.

• **Balanced Diet:** Ensure meals are balanced with lean proteins, whole grains, fruits, and vegetables to maintain stable blood sugar levels and reduce cravings.

• **Portion Control:** Use smaller plates, serve reasonable portions, and eat slowly to give your body time to feel full.

3. Practice Mindful Eating:

• **Eat Slowly and Mindfully:** Pay attention to the taste, texture, and sensations of each bite. Chew thoroughly and put down your utensils between bites.

• **Listen to Hunger Cues:** Eat when you're physically hungry, not in response to emotions or external cues like boredom or stress.

4. Manage Stress and Emotions:

• **Find Alternatives to Food:** Engage in activities that distract or relax you, such as exercise, hobbies, reading, or talking to a friend.

• **Practice Stress Management Techniques:** Deep breathing, meditation, yoga, or progressive muscle relaxation can help reduce stress without turning to food.

5. Create a Supportive Environment:

• **Stock Healthy Foods:** Keep nutritious snacks readily available and avoid keeping trigger foods in the house.

• **Seek Support:** Talk to friends, family, or a therapist about emotional eating triggers and strategies for coping.

6. Mindful Response to Cravings:

• **Delay and Distract:** When cravings strike, delay giving in for 10-15 minutes. Engage in a different activity to distract yourself and see if the craving subsides.

• **Choose Healthy Alternatives:** If you still crave a particular food, opt for a healthier version or smaller portion size.

7. Practice Self-Compassion:

• **Be Kind to Yourself:** Understand that occasional slip-ups are normal. Avoid guilt and shame, and focus on making positive choices moving forward.

8. Seek Professional Help if Needed:

• **Registered Dietitian/Nutritionist:** They can provide personalized strategies for overcoming cravings and emotional eating.

• **Therapist/Counselor:** They can help address underlying emotional issues contributing to emotional eating patterns.

9. Celebrate Non-Food Rewards:

• **Reward Yourself:** Celebrate achievements or milestones with non-food rewards, such as a massage, movie night, or a new book.

By incorporating these strategies into your daily routine and staying consistent, you can gradually reduce cravings and emotional eating behaviors, leading to a healthier relationship with food and overall well-being.

Tips For Dining Out

Dining out can present challenges for maintaining a healthy diet, but with careful planning and mindful choices, it's possible to enjoy restaurant meals without derailing your goals. Here are some tips for dining out as an endomorph or anyone looking to make healthier choices:

Before You Go:

Check the Menu Ahead of Time:

• Many restaurants now have their menus available online. Take a look beforehand to identify healthier options and plan your meal.

Eat a Healthy Snack Beforehand:

• Having a small, nutritious snack like a piece of fruit or a handful of nuts before going out can help curb excessive hunger and prevent overeating.

Stay Hydrated:

• Drink water before and during your meal to help control appetite and ensure you're not mistaking thirst for hunger.

Making Healthier Choices:

Choose Lean Proteins:

• Opt for grilled, baked, or steamed lean protein options such as chicken breast, fish, or tofu. Request sauces on the side to control portions.

Load Up on Vegetables:

• Include vegetables as much as possible. Look for salads, steamed or roasted veggies, or vegetable-based dishes.

Request Modifications:

• Don't hesitate to ask for substitutions or adjustments to suit your preferences and dietary needs. For example, swap fries for a side salad or steamed vegetables.

Portion Control:

Share or Take Half Home:

• Consider sharing a main dish with a friend or family member, or ask for a to-go box right away and portion out half of your meal before you start eating.

Mindful Eating:

• Eat slowly, savor each bite, and pay attention to your hunger and fullness cues.

This can help prevent overeating and allow you to enjoy your meal more.

Managing Desserts and Drinks:

Be Smart with Desserts:

• If you want dessert, consider sharing with others at the table or opting for a lighter option like fruit or sorbet.

Watch Beverage Choices:

• Choose water, unsweetened tea, or sparkling water instead of sugary drinks. If you choose alcohol, do so in moderation and opt for lower-calorie options.

Social and Enjoyable Dining:

Focus on Socializing:

• Enjoy the company of others and the dining experience itself rather than solely focusing on the food.

Practice Flexibility:

- Understand that dining out occasionally doesn't have to derail your progress. Aim for balance over time and avoid feelings of guilt if you indulge a bit.

After Dining Out:

Get Back on Track:

• If you indulged more than planned, resume your regular healthy eating habits with the next meal. Avoid the temptation to continue overeating due to guilt.

By implementing these tips, you can navigate dining out while maintaining a healthy diet that supports your goals as an endomorph or anyone striving for balanced nutrition and wellness. Remember, moderation and mindful choices are key to enjoying restaurant meals without compromising your health.

CHAPTER SIX
Exercise Recommendations For Endomorphs

Exercise is a crucial component for endomorphs (and everyone else) aiming to manage weight, improve metabolic health, and enhance overall fitness. Here are exercise recommendations tailored for endomorphs:

1. Combination of Cardiovascular and Strength Training:

Cardiovascular Exercise:

• Aim for at least 150 minutes of moderate-intensity aerobic exercise per week, or 75 minutes of vigorous-intensity aerobic exercise.

• Examples: Brisk walking, jogging, cycling, swimming, dancing.

• Cardio helps burn calories, improve cardiovascular health, and support weight management.

Strength Training:

• Incorporate resistance training exercises at least 2-3 times per week.

• Focus on compound exercises that target multiple muscle groups, such as squats, deadlifts, lunges, bench presses, rows, and overhead presses.

• Strength training helps build lean muscle mass, which can boost metabolism and enhance body composition.

2. Interval Training:

High-Intensity Interval Training (HIIT):

• Incorporate HIIT workouts 1-2 times per week.

• Alternating short bursts of intense exercise with recovery periods helps maximize calorie burn and improve cardiovascular fitness.

• Examples: Sprint intervals, jump squats, burpees, high knees.

3. Core Strengthening:

Core Exercises:

• Include exercises that strengthen the core muscles (abdominals, obliques, lower back).

• Examples: Planks, bicycle crunches, Russian twists, leg raises.

• A strong core supports posture, stability, and overall body strength.

4. Flexibility and Mobility:

Stretching and Mobility Work:

• Dedicate time to stretching exercises and mobility drills to improve flexibility and range of motion.

• Examples: Yoga, Pilates, dynamic stretching routines.

• Enhanced flexibility reduces the risk of injury and supports overall fitness performance.

5. Functional Training:

Functional Exercises:

• Include exercises that mimic everyday movements and improve overall functional fitness.

• Examples: Squat to press, kettlebell swings, farmer's walks, stability ball exercises.

• Functional training enhances balance, coordination, and muscular endurance.

6. Consistency and Progression:

Set Realistic Goals:

• Establish achievable fitness goals and track your progress over time.

• Gradually increase the intensity, duration, and complexity of your workouts as your fitness level improves.

7. Rest and Recovery:

Rest Days:

• Allow adequate time for rest and recovery between workouts to prevent overtraining and promote muscle repair.

• Listen to your body and adjust your exercise routine as needed based on recovery and energy levels.

8. Consultation with a Professional:

Personal Trainer or Exercise Specialist:

• Consider working with a certified personal trainer or exercise specialist, especially if you're new to exercise or need guidance on proper form and technique.

• They can tailor a workout plan to your specific needs and goals, ensuring safety and effectiveness.

By incorporating these exercise recommendations into your routine, you can effectively support weight management, improve metabolic health, and enhance overall fitness as an endomorph. Remember that consistency, variety, and enjoyment are key to sustaining a long-term exercise regimen.

Lifestyle Factors For Endomorphs

Lifestyle factors play a crucial role in managing weight, promoting overall health, and supporting metabolic balance for endomorphs. Here are key lifestyle factors that endomorphs should consider:

1. Nutrition:

• **Balanced Diet:** Focus on a balanced diet rich in whole foods, including lean proteins, complex carbohydrates, healthy fats, fruits, and vegetables.

• **Portion Control:** Monitor portion sizes to avoid overeating, especially with calorie-dense foods.

• **Meal Timing:** Aim for regular meals and snacks throughout the day to maintain stable blood sugar levels and prevent excessive hunger.

2. Physical Activity:

• **Regular Exercise:** Incorporate a combination of cardiovascular exercise (e.g., walking, jogging, cycling) and strength training (e.g., weightlifting, resistance exercises) to support metabolism, muscle development, and weight management.

• **Consistency:** Establish a consistent exercise routine and aim for at least 150 minutes of moderate-intensity aerobic activity per week, along with strength training exercises on two or more days per week.

3. Stress Management:

• **Stress Reduction Techniques:** Practice stress management techniques such as deep breathing, meditation, yoga, or mindfulness to reduce cortisol levels and support overall well-being.

• **Balance Work and Rest:** Prioritize adequate sleep (7-9 hours per night) and incorporate relaxation into your daily routine to optimize recovery and hormone balance.

4. Hydration:

• **Water Intake:** Stay hydrated by drinking plenty of water throughout the day. Limit sugary drinks and alcohol, which can contribute excess calories and affect metabolic function.

5. Mindful Eating:

• **Awareness of Eating Habits:** Practice mindful eating by paying attention to hunger and fullness cues, eating slowly, and avoiding distractions during meals.

• **Emotional Eating Awareness:** Recognize emotional triggers for eating and develop alternative coping strategies to manage emotions without turning to food.

By incorporating these lifestyle factors into your daily routine, endomorphs can effectively manage weight, support metabolic health, and improve overall well-being over the long term. Consistency, moderation, and a balanced approach are key to achieving and maintaining optimal health as an endomorph.

Supplements For Endomorphs, Safety And Effectiveness Considerations

When considering supplements for endomorphs, it's important to approach them with caution and awareness of their safety, effectiveness, and potential interactions with medications or health conditions. Here are some considerations and recommendations:

1. Safety Considerations:

• **Quality and Regulation:** Choose supplements from reputable brands that follow good manufacturing practices (GMP) and have undergone third-party testing for purity and potency.

• **Consultation:** Consult with a healthcare provider, such as a doctor or registered dietitian, before starting any new supplements, especially if you have existing health conditions or are taking medications.

• **Dosage:** Follow recommended dosages provided by healthcare professionals or as indicated on the supplement packaging. Avoid exceeding recommended doses unless advised by a healthcare provider.

2. Effectiveness Considerations:

• **Nutrient Deficiencies:** Supplements may be beneficial if you have specific nutrient deficiencies that cannot be adequately addressed through diet alone. Common deficiencies for some individuals include vitamin D, omega-3 fatty acids, and certain minerals.

• **Targeted Goals:** Choose supplements that align with your specific health goals, such as supporting metabolism, enhancing exercise performance, or improving overall nutrient intake.

3. Supplements to Consider:

• **Protein Powders:** Whey protein or plant-based protein powders can help support muscle recovery and growth, especially when combined with strength training.

• **Omega-3 Fatty Acids:** Fish oil supplements may support heart health, reduce inflammation, and potentially aid in weight management.

• **Vitamin D:** Especially important if you have limited sun exposure, vitamin D supplements can support bone health and immune function.

• **Multivitamins:** A quality multivitamin can help fill nutrient gaps in your diet, but it should not replace a balanced diet.

4. **Supplements to Approach with Caution:**

• **Weight Loss Supplements:** Be cautious of supplements marketed for rapid weight loss, as they may contain stimulants or other ingredients that can have adverse effects or interact with medications.

• **Herbal Supplements:** While some herbs have potential health benefits, they can also interact with medications or have side effects. Always research thoroughly and consult with a healthcare provider.

5. Natural Sources First:

• **Whole Foods:** Focus on obtaining nutrients from whole foods whenever possible, as they provide a balanced array of vitamins, minerals, and phytonutrients that supplements may not replicate.

• **Dietary Modifications:** Adjust your diet to include nutrient-dense foods that support your specific health needs and goals, such as lean proteins, whole grains, fruits, and vegetables.

6. Monitoring and Evaluation:

• **Track Progress:** Monitor how supplements affect your health and well-being. Discontinue use if you experience adverse effects or if they do not seem effective.

• **Regular Check-ins:** Periodically review your supplement regimen with a healthcare provider to ensure it aligns with your current health status and goals.

Supplements can be a helpful addition to support specific health goals, but they should complement a healthy diet and lifestyle rather than replace them. Always prioritize safety, consult with healthcare professionals for personalized advice, and remain mindful of your overall health and well-being as an endomorph.

Maintaining Long-Term Success

Maintaining long-term success as an endomorph involves adopting sustainable lifestyle habits that support overall health, weight management, and well-being. Here are key strategies to help you achieve and sustain your goals over time:

• **Set achievable goals** that are specific, measurable, and realistic. Break larger goals into smaller, manageable steps to track progress effectively.

• **Balanced Diet:** Emphasize whole foods such as lean proteins, whole grains, fruits, vegetables, and healthy fats. Avoid extreme diets or restrictive eating patterns that are difficult to maintain long term. Practice mindful eating and be aware of portion sizes to prevent overeating.

• **Consistent Exercise Routine:** Incorporate a variety of exercises including cardiovascular activities (e.g., walking, jogging, cycling) and strength training (e.g., weightlifting, resistance exercises). Choose activities that you find enjoyable and can sustain over time to stay motivated.

- **Stress Reduction:** Incorporate stress management techniques such as mindfulness, yoga, deep breathing, or hobbies that help you relax and unwind. Recognize triggers for emotional eating and develop alternative coping strategies that do not involve food.

- **Stay Hydrated:** Drink adequate water throughout the day to support metabolism and overall health. Aim for 7-9 hours of quality sleep per night to support recovery, hormone balance, and overall well-being.

- **Track Progress:** Keep track of your food intake, exercise routines, and how your body responds to changes. Periodically reassess your goals and make adjustments to your diet and exercise plan based on your progress and any challenges you encounter.

- **Build a Support Network:** Surround yourself with supportive friends, family members, or join a community or fitness group to stay motivated and accountable. Share your goals with others to increase motivation and receive encouragement.

• **Celebrate Successes:** Acknowledge and celebrate your achievements along the way, whether they are small or large milestones. View setbacks as opportunities to learn and grow. Identify what contributed to the setback and use it as motivation to refocus on your goals.

• **Stay Informed:** Continuously educate yourself about nutrition, fitness, and health to make informed decisions. Seek guidance from registered dietitians, nutritionists, personal trainers, or health professionals for personalized advice and support.

As an endomorph, you can achieve long-term success by integrating these strategies into your daily routine and preserving a balanced approach to health and wellness. It is crucial to maintain positive lifestyle changes over time by maintaining consistency, fortitude, and perseverance.

You can effectively manage weight, improve metabolic health, and improve overall well-being by emphasizing sustainable practices over short-term fixes. In order to promote a well-balanced diet, it is imperative to establish achievable objectives, prioritize whole foods, and exercise portion control. A variety of exercises, such as cardiovascular and strength training, can be performed to enhance fitness levels, develop lean muscle, and increase metabolism. It is essential to maintain consistency in healthy behaviors by managing stress and emotional eating through mindfulness and healthy coping strategies.

The ability to make necessary lifestyle adjustments is facilitated by the regular monitoring of progress, sufficient sleep, and hydration. Motivation and accountability are fostered by the establishment of a support network and the celebration of accomplishments along the way. Finally, it is crucial to remain informed and seek professional advice to ensure that your health journey is governed by evidence-based practices.

By adhering to these principles and adopting a sustainable approach to health and wellness, you can achieve enduring success as an endomorph and lead a more fulfilling, healthier existence.

THE END